PREFACE

This book is designed primary to supplement the students who are reading degree course in the field of Health especially in Population, Managerial Health, Economics, and Waste Management.

The student is therefore enjoined to go through the chapters very carefully to enable him/her to solve the problem in the field of Health and Waste Management.

The Co-writer, having study economics to the level of Ph.D. with the major in Economics Development for many years has identified the following major problems associated with the study of Waste Management.

Most Research on Waste Management and Disposal presented in manner confusing the student to run away from studying Health Management at the Degree level.

It is for these reasons that the writer and Co-writer deems it necessary as a young Economist to co-write this book in Waste Management & Diposal to provide a lasting solution to these problems associated with the study of Health Management.

We wish to take this opportunity to thank all my family and all my friends as well as Dr. David Ackah (Content Development Manager at Quaza Solution)

DECLARATION

I hereby declare that this dissertation is the result of my own original work and that no part of it has been presented for another degree in this university or elsewhere.

DEDICATION

To my late mother madam Margaret Antwiwaa and my dear wife Alice Aidoo and Dr. David Ackah, Content Development Manager at Quaza Solution Ltd

ACKNOWLEDGEMENTS

Coming to this far had been the contributions of some people. I wish to express my profound gratitude to my supervisor Mr. Addae Boateng Adu-Gyamfi and my head of department Prof. Akwasi Kumi-Kyereme for their constructive comments, suggestions and corrections which had helped to make this work successful. My sincere appreciation goes to Mr. Yaw Asamoah, Dauda Suleman, and my own colleague Delali for their useful advice and comments as well as to those who helped me in diverse ways to make this work successful.

Finally, I wish to extend my sincere gratitude to my friend Daniel Kono-Mantey for his encouragement and support.

ABSTRACT

Despite the high risks associated with indiscriminate disposal of solid waste, some residents in the Cape Coast Metropolis continue to bury, burn and dump refuse anywhere in their homes and surroundings without considering the health effects of their action. The study seeks to explore residents' perception, attitude and disposal practices of solid waste disposal and its health impacts in the Cape Coast Metropolis. Data for the study was obtained from two hundred and eighty - four (284) respondents. Multi-stage sampling procedure was used to generate the sample for the study. The main tool employed in gathering the data was questionnaire. The theory of planned behaviour was used to explain residents' action. The result of the study revealed that most of the respondents (75.0%) disposed of their solid waste in nearby skips with quite a number of respondents disposing their solid waste on the street. Among the solid waste disposal practices, recycling was the preferred disposal method. Forty-six per cent of the respondents expressed the opinion that the onus lies on the Metropolitan Assembly to ensure clean environments. There was a significant relationship between place of residence of respondents and their perception on solid waste disposal. It was also revealed that respondents have the perception that improper handling of solid wastes gives rise to diseases such as malaria, cholera, typhoid, diarrhoea and other respiratory tract diseases. The study recommended that the Cape Coast Metropolitan Assembly in collaboration with the Ministry of Health should intensify education on the dangers of indiscriminate dumping of solid waste.

LIST OF ACRONYMS

CCMA   Cape Coast Metropolitan Assembly

CED   Centre for Environment and Development

DESSAP   District Environmental Sanitation Strategy and Action Plan

EGSSAA   Environmental Guidelines for Small Scale Activities in Africa

MDGs   Millennium Development Goals

MLGRD   Ministry of Local Government and Rural Development

NEMA   National Environment Management Authority

OLA   Our Lady of Apostle

SEA   Strategic Environmental Assessment

UNEP   United Nations Environment Programme

UNESCO   The United Nations Educational, Scientific and Cultural Organisation

WHO   World Health Organisation

TABLE OF CONTENTS

CHAPTER ONE – INTRODUCTION 8

CHAPTER TWO – LITERATURE REVIEW 17

CHAPTER THREE - METHODOLOGY 38

CHAPTER FIVE – RESULT & DISCUSSION 49

CHAPTER FIVE – SUMMARY, CONCLUSION & RECOMMENDATION 63

REFERENCE 68

CHAPTER ONE

INTRODUCTION

Background to the Study

Issues of waste disposal have become a problem for world leaders over the years. Problems with the disposal of waste have been put forward throughout the history of human kind (Tsiboe & Marbell, 2004). Following the World Summit on Sustainable Development in Johannesburg in 2002, the United Nations General Assembly set aside the year (2008) as the "International Year of Sanitation" to raise awareness to accelerate progress towards achievement of the Millennium Development Goals (MDGs). The goal 7 specifically addresses poverty, health and other benefits that flow from better hygiene, household sanitation arrangements and waste water treatment.

Despite efforts by countries and international organisations such as the World Health Organization (WHO) to realize this goal, waste disposal which constitutes an essential aspect in household sanitation arrangement, remains an immediate and critical problem for the world. Improper disposal of solid waste pollutes the environment and poses public health hazards thereby affecting human development (Centre for Disease Control, 2009; Mills-Tettey, 2011).

Global solid waste generation in 2012, according to United Nations Environment Programme [UNEP] (2012), was 1.3 billion tonnes. This figure is estimated to rise to 2.2 billion tonnes per year by 2025, with much of the increase as a result of rapidly growing cities especially in developing countries. The UNEP indicates that low income countries are expected to generate about 213 million tonnes of solid waste a day with the population rising to about 676 million by 2025. Lower middle income countries are also projected to generate about 956 million tonnes of solid waste per day while

8

their population is projected to reach 2.08 billion by 2025 (UNEP, 2012). Moreover, waste generation is estimated to reach 360 million tonnes per day by 2025 in upper middle income countries with expected population of 619 million. For high income nations however, waste generation a day by 2025 will be about 686 million tonnes at a population of 912 million (UNEP, 2012).

In Africa, the generation of waste and its disposal; both domestic and industrial, continues to increase in cycle with growth in consumption and its association with health problems (Achankeng, 2003). For instance, per capita waste generation increased nearly three-folds over the last two decades on the continent, reaching a higher level than that in developed countries (UNEP, 2009). However, out of these huge waste generations on the continent of Africa, countries spend as much as 20 to 50 percent of their district, municipal or metropolitan revenues on waste management. Yet, two-thirds of the solid waste generated is not collected (Da Zhu et al., 2008). Such inadequate waste collection and disposal practices create problems on the environment as well as human health and consequently economic and other welfare losses. Even the collected waste ends up in an uncontrolled dump sites or burnt Achankeng, 2003 (as cited in Abagale, Mensah & Agyeman-Osei, 2012).

Although most developing countries generate solid waste far lower than developed countries, they are unable to collect the waste generated inasmuch as the developed countries which are able to collect the waste generated (Environmental Guidelines for Small Scale Activities in Africa [EGSSAA], 2009). This according to EGSSAA is generally due to poor public perception towards solid waste disposal, inadequacy of funds, fiscal irresponsibility, equipment failure, and or inadequate waste management budgets.

Various writers including Porter and Boakye-Yiadom (1997), Satterthwaite (1998) and UNEP (2005) have expressed concerns as to what has really contributed to the upsurge of improper disposal of solid waste in both developed and developing countries. Boadi and Kuitunen (2003) for instance, attributed the issue of improper disposal of solid waste to inadequacy of funding and rapid population growth especially with countries in sub-Saharan Africa. Other researchers such as Coolidge, Porter and Zhang (1998), Kendie (1998) and UNEP (2005) have also looked at solid waste problem and its relationship to increasing population growth. Taiwo (2011) attributes the issue of poor disposal of solid waste in developing countries to poverty, rapid population growth and urbanisation. This is due to fast growing rate and increasing human populations in small towns which has led to the generation of more waste.

On the contrarily, Satterthwaite (as cited in Mariwah, Kendie & Dei, 2010) argues that population growth has a positive correlation with sanitary condition, such that, fast growing cities and population growth can be associated with growing economies which make funds available for improvements in sanitary conditions. Kendie (1998) and Mariwah et al. (2010) have also argued that the increase in waste disposal problem emanates from the fact that people's perception of the essence of waste disposal issues has not been dealt with adequately. Agbola (as cited in Kendie, 1998) suggests that people's beliefs and perceptions have caused this environmental problem in many nations. This can, however, be modified or altered through education.

Contrary to Boadi and Kuitunen's (2003) argument, the United State, Environmental Protection Agency (2009) and World Health Organisation (2009) argue that the major cause of increase in solid waste has been the advent of modernization, technological advancement and increase in global population. These have created rise in demand for food and other human needs, which has also culminated into increase in the amount of waste being generated daily by individual households.

Improper solid waste disposal contributes to environmental health problems in both developed and developing countries. This is because the health implications of improper solid waste disposal can be detrimental to people exposed to such situations especially school children, waste workers, and workers in facilities producing toxic and contagious material. Other high-risk groups include population living near a waste dump and those, whose water supply has become contaminated due to either waste dumping or leakage from landfill sites. Uncollected solid waste also increases risk of injury and infection (Danso-Manu, 2011).

Moreso, it is estimated that in Africa about 70 per cent outpatient cases are sanitation and environmental related diseases (MLGRD, 2010). Consequently, improper solid waste disposal have a very high economic and social cost in the public health services, as has been estimated by governments, industries, and families (Abul, 2010).

The issue of solid waste cannot be exhausted without looking at its management in some countries. Senkoro (2003) argues that waste management is the world second problem after the problem of unemployment. Despite the formulation of Waste Management Regulation in 2006 by African Countries including Kenya which aims to streamline the handling, transportation and disposal of various types of waste, different kinds of waste are still dumped in an uncontrolled manner with hazardous waste seriously poisoning the environment which endangers the health of both humans and animals (NEMA, 2012). This is as a result of poor perception of people towards solid waste handling and disposal in developing countries (Addo, 2010).

Perception plays an important role in the generation, disposal and overall disposal of solid waste. Dango, Zurbrugg, Cisse, Obrist, Tanner and Biemi (2010) in a study conducted in Abidjan indicated that people in poor settlements had low levels of awareness of health implications of solid waste disposal. They therefore had negative perceptions towards handling of solid waste and the negative health implications therein. Sessa, Giuseppe, Marinelli and Angelillo (2009) in a study conducted in Italy also observed that residents with low levels of education, however, perceived indiscriminate disposal of solid waste as associated with health problems. Sessa et al. (2009) therefore argued that education does not necessarily influence perceptions towards solid waste disposal. Longe, Longe and Ukpebor (2009) on the other hand indicated that education of residents plays a major role in their perceptions and attitudes towards household solid waste disposal. They thus argued that low levels of education negatively influence perception of people towards solid waste disposal.

The problem of solid waste disposal in Ghana is the same as those faced in other parts of the world (Mensah & Larbi, 2005). Ghana is witnessing a population explosion in its towns and cities, and sanitation related inadequacies contributing to poor health are the predisposing issues in a high percentage of diseases reported (Boadi & Kuitunen, 2005). Also, the United Nations Human Development Report of 2008 indicates that 15,000 children die in Ghana annually due to sanitation related diseases before attaining the age of five.

Though, waste management has been outsourced or franchised to some private companies such as Zoomlion Ghana Limited, there is the problem of delay in lifting public containers and littering around which obstruct rain water runoff, resulting in the forming of stagnant water bodies that serve as breeding grounds for vectors which cause diseases (Tsiboe & Marbell, 2004). Not discounting the above practices, other factors might have compounded the problem. People's perceptions towards solid waste disposal must therefore not be overlooked.

Like other cities in Ghana, Cape Coast is faced with solid waste disposal problem both in open and enclosed areas in the Metropolis

(Strategic Environmental Assessment, 2010). This is because the Metropolis has challenges with solid waste from generation, through storage and treatment to disposal posing health problems to the people in the Metropolis. Residents' perception of solid waste disposal therefore, needs to be unravelled. There is therefore the need to research into residents' perceptions of solid waste disposal.

Statement of the problem

Cape Coast Metropolis generates about 241.8 tonnes of solid waste daily. Out of this about 184 tonnes representing 76 per cent is collected and disposed at the final disposal site. The remaining 57.8 tonnes (24%) is indiscriminately disposed leading to the creation of unsightly "waste hills" in several locations of the metropolis thereby threatening the health of the population (CCMA-DESSAP, 2009). Increasing amounts of waste emanating from residential, commercial and industrial areas and their poor management are results from poor planning of waste management programmes, inadequate budgetary support from government and negative attitudes and perceptions towards waste (CCMA-DESSAP, 2009).

Although the Cape Coast Metropolitan Assembly (CCMA) has made significant efforts to addressing the solid waste disposal situation some residents do not dispose refuse into containers that have been provided. Even those who make the attempt to take their refuse to these containers some discard it on the ground rather than into the containers. In some communities in the metropolis (for instance, Abura and Pedu) residents bury their refuse due to their negative attitudes and perceptions towards solid waste disposal (Addo, 2010).

In some parts of the metropolis, solid waste is disposed improperly (personal observation). These in effect, have negative health implications for some residents of the metropolis. Records from the Cape Coast Metropolitan

Health Directorate reveal that about 70 per cent of reported outpatient cases are sanitation-related diseases, of which malaria accounts for 53% of reported cases in the metropolis (Ghana Health Service, Cape Coast, 2012).

Much research has been conducted on solid waste disposal. Boadi and Kuitunen (2003), for instance, investigated municipal solid waste management in Accra metropolitan area in Ghana. Cointreau (1982) studied the environmental management of urban solid wastes in developing countries while Danso-Manu (2011) assessed the nature of solid waste disposal in Ghana with emphasis on data collection for good management practices; Addo (2010) studied the waste disposal practices and management in Cape Coast and Kendie (1998) explored residents' attitudes towards waste disposal in Cape Coast. It appears much attention has not been given to residents' perception of solid waste disposal in Ghana.

Objectives of the study

The main objective of the study was to assess residents' perception of solid waste disposal in the Cape Coast Metropolis. Specifically, the study sought to;
1. Identify solid waste disposal practices of residents in the Metropolis;
2. Assess attitudes of residents towards solid waste disposal;
3. Analyse the perceptions of residents on Solid waste disposal and;
4. Discuss residents' perceived health implications of disposal of solid waste.

Research Questions

The study sought to provide answers to the following research questions
1. What are the solid waste disposal practices among residents of Cape Coast Metropolis?

2. What are the attitudes of residents of Cape Coast Metropolis towards solid waste disposal?

3. How do residents perceive about solid waste disposal situation in the Metropolis?

4. What are the perceived health implications of solid waste disposal?

Hypothesis

H0: there is no significant relationship between place of residence and disposal practices.

H0: there is no significance difference in the perception of residents and health problems associated with solid waste disposal.

Significance of the study

The study is significant in many ways. This study adds to the existing knowledge on solid waste disposal and most particularly unearthing new approaches in dealing with people's perception on solid waste disposal and its health implications in the country and worldwide. The findings would also help Cape Coast Metropolitan Assembly to organise better sanitation and hygiene educational programmes for residents and desensitise their perceptions towards solid waste disposal.

It will also increase the awareness on issues relating to waste disposal for the Metropolis and policy makers especially at the local level. Finally, the study forms a baseline study to which future studies can be compared to keep track of changing perceptions of residents towards solid waste disposal in the Cape Coast Metropolis.

Organization of the Study

The study was divided into five chapters. Chapter One covered the background of the study, the statement of problem, objectives of the study, research questions, significance of the study and the organization of the study. Chapter Two dealt with the literature review of existing work in the subject area. The third Chapter involved the methodology used in the study. Chapter Four dealt with the results of the study and discussions of the study while chapter Five looked at the summary, conclusions and recommendations.

CHAPTER TWO
LITERATURE REVIEW

Introduction

This chapter reviews literature relevant to the study. The review of the literature is divided into two sections; Theoretical and Conceptual Frameworks. The theoretical framework reviews general empirical literature relevant to the study. These include waste, types of solid waste, solid waste disposal practices, generation of solid waste, perception of solid waste disposal, attitude towards solid waste disposal and perceived health implications of solid waste disposal; and the conceptual framework to underpin the study.

Definition of waste Concepts are sometimes seen as foundations of communication which are abstracted from perceptions and are used to convey and transmit information (Nachmias & Nachmias 1996). Despite the fact that much has been done about waste worldwide, the definition of waste is quite rare in scholarly literature (Achor, Ehikwe & Nwafor, 2014). The term "wastes" according to the World Bank (2000) is defined as "useless, un-used, un-wanted or discarded materials" (p. 2). Waste can also be defined as any material having no direct value to the producer and so must be disposed of. The entire concept of wastes is subject to the value judgment of the primary owner or potential consumer (Davies, 2004). Waste is therefore viewed as a discarded material which has no consumption value to the person abandoning it. Wastes include solids, liquids and gases (U.S.E.P.A, 2009). The gaseous wastes are principally industrial fumes and smoke; while the liquefied wastes consist mainly of sewage and the fluid part of industrial wastes. Solid wastes on the other hand, are very often classified as refuse. Solid waste is therefore synonymous with refuse. Refuse is generated from several sources. It can be generated from domestic activities such as cooking, sweeping, cleaning, fuel burning and gardening (Cointreau, 2002). According to Cointreau (2002) other sources of solid wastes generation are the industries, the commercial areas like markets, various institutions such as schools, hospitals, government offices, barracks, and agricultural activities.

Dijkema, Reuter and Verhoef (2000) assert that waste is a subjective concept and that what is considered waste presently, may become a resource in the future because ''waste'' has not been put to its full potential use. As noted by Moeller (2005), the term is frequently left undefined due to its varied definition. As a default definition, Moeller (2005) suggests that any substance that is without an owner is waste. In spite of its critical importance a list of types of waste is frequently substituted for the underlying definition.

Definitions of waste are rather commonly found in such documents as dictionaries, encyclopaedia, technical reports of governments, and organizations. For example, Gadsby (2003) defines waste as "the unwanted material or substance that is left after you have used something" (p.1612). This means that when something or substance is no longer in use it can be referred to as waste.   Maurice (2007) on the other hand defines waste as "the unusable material left over from a process of manufacture, the use of consumer goods, or the useless by-products of a process" (Maurice , 2007, P. 2345).

Abduli and Nasrabadi (2007) however provide a more elaborate definition of the term waste. According to them the concept of waste embraces all unwanted and economically unusable by-products or residuals at any given place and time, and any other matter that may be discarded accidentally or otherwise into the environment. Abduli and Nasrabadi (2007) further suggest that what constitutes waste must occur in such a volume,

18

concentration, constituency or manner as to cause a significant alteration in the environment. Thus, apart from waste being an unwanted substance that is discarded, the amount of it and the impact it makes on the environment also become important considerations in defining waste.

Markwara (2011) also referred to waste as the unwanted materials arising entirely from human activities which are discarded into the environment. They further argued that there is no constellation of properties inherent in any lump, object or material which will serve to identify it as waste. The notion that waste results entirely from human activities is corroborated by Jessen (2002) who noted that waste is human creation and "there is no such thing as waste in nature where cut-offs of one species become food for another" (Jessen, 2002, p.78). As noted by Jessen, our waste stream is actually full of resources going in the wrong direction.

An item according to Kistner (2005) becomes waste when the holder or owner does not wish to take further responsibility for it. Davies (2008) also describes waste as "unwanted or unusable materials that emanate from numerous sources from industry and agriculture as well as businesses and households and can be liquid, solid or gaseous in nature, and hazardous or non-hazardous depending on its location and concentration" (Davies, 2008, p. 4). Davies further noted that "what some people consider to be waste materials or substances are considered a source of value by others". This relative attribute of waste can be compared with the concept of "resource" which has also been defined as material that has use-value (Barlaz, Kaplan, Ranjithan & Rynk, 2003). Just as a material becomes a resource when it gains use-value, it also becomes waste when it loses its use-value. Like resources, waste is also a relative concept or human appraisal because what constitutes waste can vary from one person to another, one society to another and over time (Barlaz et al., 2003).

Deducing from the views expressed above, the definition of waste to be used in this study is any solid substance discarded into the environment because it is unwanted, which causes significant nuisance or adverse impact in the environment and the health of the inhabitants living in that environment.

Types of solid waste

Solid waste is the term used to describe non-liquid waste material arising from domestic, trade, commercial, agricultural, industrial, and public services through human activities. The quantity and composition of some types of solid wastes vary from day to day, season to season and from locality to locality. Operationally, it can be said that, solid waste is any material which comes from domestic, commercial, and industrial sources arising from human activities which has no value to people who possess it and is discarded as useless. Solid waste may be classified as domestic (residential) waste, clinical waste, commercial waste, metropolitan waste, institutional waste, construction and demolition waste, sanitation waste and industrial waste (UNEP, 2007).

Domestic or household waste according to Kendie (2003) arises from homes and also includes refuse or rubbish from schools. This form of waste as argued by UNEP (2007) mainly involves packaging papers, plastics, textiles, glass, metals, putrescible materials, newsprint and food leftovers. Kendie (2003) indicated that clinical waste is the waste that arises from medical, nursing, dental, veterinary and pharmaceutical investigation, teaching and research. UNEP (2007) argues that this waste includes human or animal tissue, drugs or pharmaceutical products, swabs, dressings, syringes, needles or sharp instruments. This type of solid waste is usually harmful when one comes into contact with them unless rendered safe (Kendie, 2003).

Rushbrook and Pugh (1999) wrote that commercial waste includes waste from shops, offices, restaurants, hotels and similar commercial establishments. The waste typically consists of packaging materials, office supplies, food wastes and has a close similarity to some components of domestic waste. In lower-income countries food markets may contribute to a large proportion of this type of waste.

Metropolitan waste according to Centre for Environment and Development (CED) (2003), includes wastes such as street sweeping, roadside litter, litter from municipal dustbins, dead animals and abandoned vehicles. Metropolitan waste includes rubbish, trash and almost all types of waste.

Rushbrook and Pugh (1999) described institutional waste produced in establishments such as government offices, schools, hospitals and other healthcare facilities, military bases and religious buildings. The waste generally includes components similar to both domestic and commercial waste (Moeller, 2005). Hospital wastes as argued by Moeller include potentially hazardous, infectious and pathological materials such as used bandages, sharp objects including syringes, needles and items contaminated with body fluids including blood. It is important to separate the hazardous and non-hazardous fractions in healthcare waste to reduce the risk to health and pollution.

Waste from demolished buildings and other structures are classified, according to CED (2003), as demolition waste. Waste from the construction, remodelling and repairing of individual residences, housing complexes, multi-stored flats, commercial buildings etc. are classified construction wastes. The constituents of this waste are stores, concrete, bricks, plaster and plumbing.

Rushbrook and Pugh (1999) indicate that in several lower-income countries no sewage network exists within many towns to remove faeces and similar solid sanitation wastes. Specialised collectors of night soil often collect this waste separately from individual houses. This material, according to Swan (2003), can contaminate watercourses and become a source of infectious diseases if indiscriminately dumped. Rushbrook and Pugh (1999) argue that in those cities where there are no sewage treatment facilities for night soil, it is common for this material to be used either for manure for agricultural crops or end up at the metropolitan landfill.

Kendie (2003) described industrial waste as involving materials or substances that come from industries. Such waste according to Kendie may be hazardous, toxic or ordinary. This includes empty oil containers and scraps. Agricultural waste includes waste that arises from agricultural practices or activities. This includes silage liquors, straw, plant stems, farm slurry that is often sprayed on farm as liquid manure and containers used for fertilizers and pesticides.

Solid waste disposal practices

Several disposal practices have changed over the years. These practices according to the Centre for Environment and Development (2003) vary greatly with types of wastes and local conditions. In the contemporary era, the disposal practices include recycling, composting, landfilling and incineration (Centre for Environment and Development, 2003). These practices are explained below:

Recycling

Kitbuah, Asase, Yusif, Mensah & Fischer, (2009) wrote that waste reduction can be accomplished through the increased use of source separation and subsequent material recovery and recycling. According to Kitbuah et al. (2009) separating waste materials at the household level occurs to some extent almost universally, and prevents the most valuable and reusable materials from being discarded. Following in-home retention of valuable materials, Gyankumah (2004) indicated that waste-pickers usually remove most valuable materials either before garbage enters the waste stream or en route, especially in the lower and middle income areas of many municipalities. To be effective, Abul (2010) argues that policies need to be implemented on both the national and local levels.

Composting

The waste of many nations according to Hester and Harrison (2003) would theoretically be ideal for reduction through composting, having a much higher composition of organic material than industrialized countries. In developing countries, the average city's municipal waste stream is over (50%) organic material (Hester & Harrison, 2003). Although well documented in China and other areas of Eastern Asia, composting projects as argued by UNEP (2007) have had a spotty record throughout Africa, Latin America and elsewhere, and have had the largest number of failed facilities worldwide. According to Olar (2003), composting significantly reduces the amount of waste requiring ultimate disposal, extending the life of landfills and also has the potential of increasing soil fertility. In the view of Mensa (2011) most developing countries which have found success with composting have found that it works best when implemented at the household and community levels.

Land filling

The placement of solid waste in landfills is probably the oldest and definitely the most prevalent form of ultimate garbage disposal (Palczynski, 2004). Dolk (2003) found varying amounts of planning and engineering in

Municipal Solid Waste dumping; among the various regions visited, African nations (with the exception of South Africa) had the fewest engineered landfills, with most nations practicing open dumping for waste disposal.

Moeller (2005) outlined four features that must be present in order for a landfill to be considered sanitary: Full or partial hydro geological isolation through the use of liners to prevent leachate infiltration into the soil and groundwater. In addition, there should also be formal engineering preparations with an examination of geological and hydrological features as well as permanent control, with trained and equipped staff to supervise construction and use. There should also be planned waste emplacement and covering. Swan (2003) observed that there are naturally few people who would be excited by having a landfill in their backyard.

Incineration

Despite the fact that incineration is a solid waste disposal practice, Olar (2003) argues that it should not be considered a disposal option. This method leads to the dispersal of some ash and constituent chemicals into the atmosphere. Gyankumah (2004) however stated that, with occasional exceptions, incineration is an inappropriate technology for most low-income countries. Above all, the high financial start-up and operational capital required to implement incineration facilities according to UNEP (2006) is a major barrier to successful adoption in developing countries.

Browne and Allen (2007) indicated that transportation of waste to select centralized sanitary landfills, instead of open dumps on each island, could be prohibitively expensive and time consuming. Being surrounded by open water increases the attractiveness of ocean dumping. Reduction by incineration, along with sanitary disposal of the residue, would be a useful alternative to traditional disposal methods, and have proven useful in nations such as Bermuda and the British Virgin Islands (Browne & Allen, 2007).

Burying

In urban cities, solid waste are disposed of indiscriminately in any available space without care of health and environmental impacts associated with it (Mbalisi & Offor, 2012). Boadi & Kuitunen (2005) also confirmed that burying of solid waste poses both environmental and health threats through pollution and breeding of pathogenic organisms. They further indicated that burying which are practised by many individuals are not environmentally friendly because they aid in the spreading of diseases and the pollution of the environment. Many studies have attributed burying of solid waste to inadequate waste facilities (Boadi & Kuitunen, 2005). Study by Babayemi and Dauda (2009) in Nigeria confirmed that burying had the highest percentage (64.2%) among all the disposal practices. Residents cited unavailability of waste containers as the reason for their action .

However, Chati (2012) in a study conducted in Saboba also observed that about 70 percent of respondents bury their solid waste although there were adequate communal skips. Hamdi (2003) indicated that good solid waste devoid of burying has to do with changing behaviour and habits.

Indiscriminate dumping

Indiscriminate dumping of solid waste result inadequate waste facilities which threatens the health of residents (Boadi & Kuituinen, 2005). According to Malombe (1993) irregular services by municipal councils compel people to practice indiscriminate dumping. Studies by Benneh et al. (1993) in Ghana indicated that about 83 percent of Ghanaians practice indiscriminate dumping. This according to them was as a result of their weak capacity to handle solid waste. Consequently, Nze (1978) attributed indiscriminate dumping to lack of logistics and financial management and people's attitudes towards waste management. Sule (1981) also observed indiscriminate dumping can be ascribed to improper management of solid wastes and the lack of seriousness in the enforcement of bye-laws governing solid waste disposal. Moreover, Karley (1993) attributed Ghana's problem of indiscriminate dumping to lack of suitable site for solid waste. consequently, studies by Benneh et al (1993) reveal that residents in low-income areas practice indiscriminate dumping; this is because they are not served with adequate waste facilities. Boadi and Kuitunnen (2005) also indicated that indiscriminate dumping is high among households that store solid waste in plastic bags. The conclusion one can make here is that burying and indiscriminate dumping of solid waste may be as a result of unavailable waste facilities in residents' locality. This makes residents dispose of refuse indiscriminately without looking at the health risk that it poses.

Explanation of perception

The word perception has been defined by different scholars. Bartley (2009) states that perception is the immediate discriminatory response of the organism to energy activating sense organs. To Fieandt (2006) perception is an experienced sensation that is a phenomenal impression resulting functionally from certain inputs. Also, Forgus (2010) adds that perception is the process by which an organism receives or extracts certain information about the environment.

Similarly, Barnhart (2008) explains that perception is the state of being aware of something through the senses that is, to see, hear, taste, smell, and feel. It also involves insights, apprehension, discrimination and comprehension. Finally, Melissa (2002) sees perception as a particular way of understanding or thinking about something. From the above definitions, it can be deduced that the word perception is how people react to a phenomenon (solid waste disposal) in their community. To add to that perception deals with one's awareness, understanding, interpretation and impression made by others and knowledge of a situation or a phenomenon. To conclude, Perception is subjective and it varies from person to another. This is due to how perceptual systems are structured and how individuals "see" things in terms of knowledge, beliefs and expectations.

Perception of solid waste disposal

Perception of people plays a major role in solid waste disposal, in that if people have negative perception about solid waste disposal, little or no attention will be given to it and vice versa. Perceptions may be positively influenced through awareness building, sensitisation and education about the negative aspects of inadequate waste collection with regard to public health (Bernstein, 2004). As noted by (Gyankumah, 2004), efforts to address solid waste disposal problems in developing countries, have failed due to the negative perception people have towards solid waste disposal. Banjo, Adebambo and Dairo (2009) in their study conducted on the perception of the inhabitants of Ijebu-ode on domestic waste disposal noted that about 50 per cent of the respondents disposed their domestic wastes once in a week. Larger part of the waste observed included cans, plastic products, polythene bags, food materials green wastes, bottles and paper.

Domestic waste, when sorted and treated well according to Franduah (2008), can be turned into a resource but the greater part of waste generated in Ijebu-Ode as argued by Banjo, Adebambo and Dairo (2009) seemed not to have undergone any sorting or treatment before the final disposal. They were left as indicated by Banjo et al. (2009) in piles for weeks and kept in or around houses most especially closer to kitchens to create unsanitary scenes that produces offensive odour and, worst of all create diseases like cholera and typhoid fever. This therefore indicates that the inhabitants do not perceive improper handling of solid waste as having any negative health implication. These arguments are confirmed by Franduah's (2008) study in which he noted that the greater percentage of waste storing containers in Nima were sacks and that none of this storing containers had cover, the implications of which are negative health consequences. The conclusion one can make here is that residents' negative perception towards waste makes them dispose of refuse indiscriminately without looking at the health risk that it poses.

Perceptions toward health implication of solid waste disposal

While Abul (2010) defines perception as an individual's understanding of something or someone, Adekunle, Oguns, Shekwolo, Igbuku and Ogunkoya (2012) terms perception as a way of regarding, understanding or interpreting something, a mental impression of a given phenomenon. Residents' perception plays an important role in shaping the relationship between their health and environment. Ferner (as cited in Njagi et al., 2013) argues that relationships between an environmental contaminant and health are the results of the perceptions that an individual has been exposed to, which in turn are influenced by a host of individual and contextual factors such as environment and attitudes. People's perception regarding the health implications of solid waste disposal is duly influenced by the settings that they find themselves and their general upbringing.

Mosquera-Becerra, Gomez-Gutierrez, Mendez-paz (2009) argue that even though people in developing countries hold the perception that improper solid waste disposal results in negative health outcomes yet, their unfavourable economic conditions do not permit them to deal with the solid waste disposal problems. For instance, many of them including Ghana depend on donor support from countries and international organizations such as the United States of America and the World Bank, to finance their yearly financial budgets. Sessa, Giuseppe, Marinelli, Angelillo (2009) however indicate that people generally perceive health implications of improper solid waste disposal lightly, and do generally little to tackle the situation. Sessa et al. (2009) attribute the low perceptions of people towards negative health outcomes associated with disposal of solid waste to low levels of education. Sessa et al. (2009) also noted that people with higher levels of formal education however perceive the negative health outcomes of improper solid waste disposal highly and appreciate the relationships that exist between solid waste disposal and health. They therefore put in measures at the individual level to deal with the situation. Such measures include provision of dustbins at their places of residence and separation of solid waste before disposal.

Attitude towards solid waste disposal

Attitude is an enduring predisposition towards a particular aspect of one's environment (McDougal & Munro, 1987 as cited in Mariwah 2010). According to Warner (no date as cited in Mariwah) attitude consists of three basic components which include perception (emotional impression), cognition (thought) and behavioural tendency to act.

Bowersox, Closs and Cooper, (2005) argue that waste generation is conditioned to an important degree by people's attitudes towards waste: their patterns of material use and waste handling, their interest in waste reduction and minimisation, the degree to which they separate wastes and the extent to which they refrain from indiscriminate dumping and littering. People's attitudes influence not only the characteristics of waste generation, but also the effective demand for waste collection services, in other words, their interest in and willingness to pay for collection services (Bowersox et al., 2005).

Attitude towards solid waste disposal, according to Browne and Allen (2007) may be positively influenced through awareness-building campaigns and educational measures on the negative impacts of inadequate waste collection with regard to public health and environmental conditions, and the value of effective disposal. Thrift (2007) however suggests that such campaigns should inform people of their responsibilities as waste generators and of their rights as citizens to waste management services.

While attitude towards solid waste maybe positively influenced by public information and educational measures, improved waste handling patterns can hardly be maintained in the absence of practical waste disposal options (Bowersox et al., 2005). Awareness-building measures as noted by Johansson (2006) should therefore be coordinated with improvements in waste collection services, whether public or community-managed. Similarly, people's waste generation and disposal patterns are influenced by those of their neighbours. A collective logic is involved because improved waste handling practices will only yield significant environmental impacts if most households in an area participate in the improvement (Johansson, 2006). Besides general awareness, improved local waste management depends upon the availability of practical options for waste collection anda consensus among neighbours that improvements are both important and possible (Thrift, 2007).

Kaseva and Mbuligwe (2003) suggest that industrial establishments present special problems regarding waste disposal patterns due to the volume and /or the occasionally hazardous nature of the generated wastes. Regulation and control measures should be employed as far as possible. Thrift (2007) however argues that these measures are seldom very effective as is often the case. Public awareness, reliable service options and consensus are crucial to improving waste generation and disposal patterns of industrial enterprises (Kaseva & Mbuligwe, 2003).

The negative attitude for solid waste disposal can be more practicable in Ghana and the study area in particular where solid waste disposal issue is no one's business and it is somebody's work attitude among residents (if I don't litter somebody will not get work to do).

Health implications of solid waste disposal

According to Abul (2010) solid waste disposal sites are usually found on the outskirts of urban areas, turning into the child sources of contamination due to the incubation and proliferation of flies, mosquitoes and rodents which in turn are disease transmitters that negatively affect health. Mizpah and Jay (2009) indicate that dumpsites are known for their smelly and unsightly conditions in many countries especially in developing ones. These conditions according to Abul (2010) are worse in rainy seasons because of extreme temperatures which speed up the rate of bacterial action on biodegradable organic materials.

Most developing countries, like Swaziland, use such dumpsites rather than properly managed and environmentally safe landfills. Mazmanian and Kraft (2005) noted that lack of capital and poor government policies regarding solid waste contribute to such conditions. There is therefore considerable public concern over the possible effects of dumpsites on the health of people living nearby, particularly those where hazardous waste is dumped (Mazmanian & Kraft, 2005). Disposal of solid waste on the land without careful planning and management can present a danger to the environment and the human health (Mizpah & Jay, 2009).

Moeller (2005) suggests that there are potential risks to health from improper handling of solid waste. Direct health implications concern mainly the workers in this field, who need to be protected, as far as possible, from contact with waste. There are also specific risks in handling wastes from hospitals and clinics. For the general public, the main risks to health are

31

indirect and arise from the breeding of disease vectors, primarily flies and rats (Hester & Harrison, 2003). The study area (Cape Coast) has similar characteristics where top ten diseases in the metropolis is sanitation – related.

Uncontrolled hazardous wastes from industries mixing up with municipal wastes according to UNEP (2007) create potential negative implications to human health. Traffic accidents as noted by Swan (2003) result from toxic spilled wastes. Browne and Allen (2007) argue that there is specific danger of concentration of heavy metals in the food chain. According to Browne and Allen (2007) such a problem illustrates the relationship between solid waste and liquid industrial effluents containing heavy metals discharged into drainage/sewerage systems and/or open dumping sites of municipal/metropolitan solid wastes. Browne and Allen (2007) indicate that the wastes discharged thereby maintain a vicious cycle of negative health implications including chemical poisoning through chemical inhalation, uncollected waste obstructing the storm, water runoff resulting in flood, low birth weight, cancer, congenital malformations, neurological disease, nausea and vomiting.

Goorah, Esmyot and Boojhawon (2009) however argue that health implications of solid waste disposal include exposure to toxic chemicals through air, water and soil media; exposure to infection and biological contaminants; stress related to odour, noise, vermin and visual amenity; risk of fires, explosions, and subsidence; spills, accidents and transport emissions.

Roel, Eddy and Thierry (2010) wrote that the major practices adopted in disposing waste have their various health implications. Health implications of composting for instance include noise, odour and unsightliness. Additionally, many of the micro-organisms found in compost are known respiratory sensitizers that can cause a range of respiratory symptoms including allergic rhinitis, asthma, and chronic bronchitis (Appiah, Obeng, Donkor & Mensah, 2009). Composting according to Roel et al. (2010) is aerobic and produces primarily carbon dioxide, while anaerobic digestion produces methane. Both gases contribute to global warming (Appiah et al., 2009).

Poku (2009) states that the most serious health implication of incineration as a solid waste disposal practice is from air emissions, which include particulates, CO, NOx, acid gases (chlorides and sulfides), volatile organics and mercury. These compounds contribute to bioaccumulation of toxics and acid rain. Inhalation of particulate matter poses a health danger: smaller particles are more likely to carry heavy metals, which run can be retained in lung tissue and enter the bloodstream (Scheinberg, Anschutz & Van de, 2006).

Health implications of landfills according to UNEP (2007) include odour nuisance; ozone formation (from reaction of Nitrogen Oxide and non-methane organic compounds with sunlight) that cause pulmonary and central nervous system damage; fire and explosion hazards from build-up of methane; an increase in the number of vermin (birds, rodents and insects) which act as disease vectors; and ground and air pollution from leachate and landfill gases. Gladding (2004) stated that recycling as a solid waste disposal method also has health implications. Sorting facilities contain high concentrations of dust, bio-aerosols and metals. Workers commonly experience itching eyes, sore throats, and respiratory diseases (Gladding, 2004).

According to the UNEP, 2007 depending on the source of solid waste; industrial waste example, fall off or unused chemicals and raw materials, expired products and substandard goods; agricultural waste example, pesticides (herbicides and fungicides); hospital waste, example, packaging materials and containers, used syringes and sharps, biological waste and

33

pharmaceuticals there are varied health implications of the disposal of solid waste materials in human health. These health implications according to the UNEP include; skin disorders-fungal infection, allergic dermatitis, pruritis and skin cancer; respiratory abnormalities-bacterial upper respiratory tract infections and other health diseases related to sanitation.

Income and solid waste disposal

It is perceived generally that people with low income levels degrade the environment by practising improper solid waste disposal practices (Murad, Hasan & Rahman, 2012). They further explain that households with low levels of income are willing to practice proper waste disposal but their economic hardship force them to dispose indiscriminately. However, Murad, Hasan & Rahman (2012) in their study in Jinjang Utara found that low-income households generate lower waste per person than middle and high income households. Therefore, low income groups contribute much less to environmental degradation caused by their poor waste disposal. Afroz et al. (2010) ; Sivakumar & Sugirtharan, (2010) and Medina (2002) also observed a significant relationship between a community's income and the amount of solid waste generated. This means that high and middle income households generate high amount of waste. Waste generation and its disposal is greatly influenced by household's level of income.

Study by Bandara et al. (2007) on household income and types of waste generated noted that organic waste and waste separation is high among household with high levels of income. This may imply that high income household could afford plenty waste bins for different waste generated.

Conceptual Framework

This part talks about the conceptual framework that will guide the study. It describes the nature and characteristics of behaviour and perception of people as well as the application of the framework to issues related to waste disposal. In order to explain residents' perception towards solid waste, the theory of Planned Behaviour was adopted.

Theory of Planned Behaviour

The Theory of Planned Behaviour was propounded by Ajzen in the year 2002 to explain human action. The theory has been applied successfully in a number of areas such as healthy eating, hunting, leisure choice, travel mode, unethical behaviour, waste management and recycling. In this study however, solid waste disposal is the focus. According to Ajzen (2002) human behaviour is guided by three kinds of consideration. These are beliefs about the likely outcomes of the behaviour and the evaluations of these outcomes (behavioural beliefs), beliefs about the normative expectations of others and motivation to comply with these expectations (normative beliefs), and beliefs about the presence of factors that may promote or hinder the performance of the behaviour (control beliefs). With regards to solid waste, if residents hold positive beliefs about solid waste disposal, it will influence them to exhibit positive attitudes towards solid waste disposal and thereby promoting good health.

The three considerations; attitude towards the behaviour (good disposal practices), norms, perceptions and values of behavioural control, thus guide a person to form a behavioural intention such as proper disposal of solid waste which helps promote the health of residents.

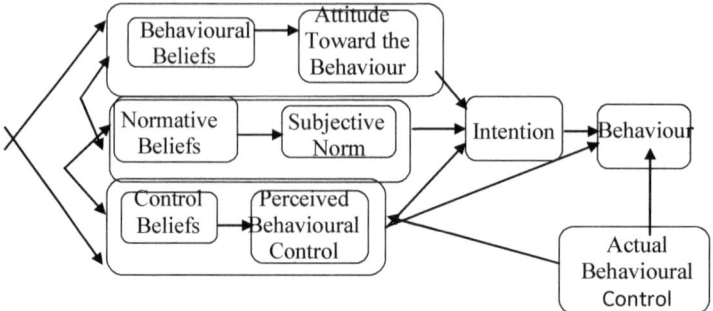

Figure 1: Theory of Planned Behaviour

Source: Ajzen (2002)

This framework is relevant to this study because one perception are influenced by his knowledge, beliefs, values and norms which one can get without experience and knowledge of the person.   Moreover, the more knowledge one has about handling solid waste, the clearer one's perceptions towards good sanitation tends to be, and the stronger and better one's attitudes towards handling of solid waste. The theory of Planned Behaviour however has its focus on behaviour neglecting other aspect such as awareness and knowledge to affect a change. This is where Pred Behavioural Matrix Model play a role in this study to strengthen its weaknessess.

Pred's Behavioural Matrix

Information constitutes an important element for bringing awareness and knowledge upon which good solid disposal practice can be made. Hence to analyse the knowledge and attitudes of residents towards proper solid waste disposal, the Pred's (1967) Behavioural matrix informed the study (Figure 2). Pred's posits that a decision-making situation is a function of the quantity and quality of information available in a given environment. That is, the readiness of residents to practice proper solid waste disposal depends on the quantity and quality of information they have regarding proper waste disposal.

For example, if residents have poor quality information about solid waste disposal such as waste are not harmful or dirty environment cannot make them sick, then they will practice improper waste disposal, irrespective of their educational level. The model again explains that some residents may make good use of the quality of information based on the quality of information they have (Bnn).

However, those residents without quality information may not be able to make rational decisions (B11, B 12, B13). On the other hand, others may not have adequate information but would be able to make rational decisions (B1n, B2n) whilst others may obtain optimal information but make irrational decisions (Bn1, Bn2, Bn3). According to Pred, in between these groups are a countless of combinations of decision makers based on the quality and quantity of information available to them.

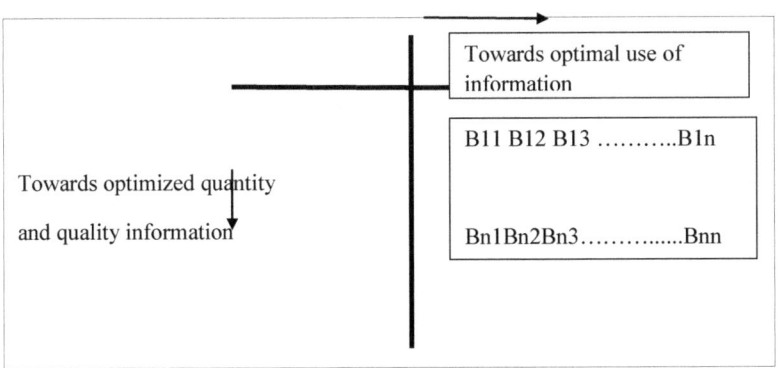

Source: Pred (1967)

The model is useful in examining the quality and quantity of information available to people regarding solid waste disposal situation in their locality.

CHAPTER THREE
METHODOLOGY
Introduction

This chapter explains in detail the methodology employed to collect the necessary data for the study. It covers the study area, research design, target population, sample size, sampling procedure, research instruments, data collection procedure and analysis.

Study area

The study area is Cape Coast Metropolitan Area (Figure 1) in the Central Region of Ghana. It is one of the two hundred and sixteen (216) administrative districts in Ghana. It serves as both a district capital of the Cape Coast Metropolitan Area as well as Administrative capital of the Central Region. The metropolis was the first national capital of the then Gold Coast (now Ghana). The removal of the seat of Government to Accra in 1877 marked the beginning of the economic decline of Cape Coast, a trend that has continued to date. Cape Coast which used to be the third largest town in Ghana in 1960 declined to the sixth in 1970, the ninth in 1984 and the tenth in 2000 (Kendie, 1998).

Population

The population growth rate of Cape Coast which was 1.8 per cent between 1970 and 1984 reduced to 1.39 per cent between 1984 and 2000 and then increased to 2.1 per cent between 2000 and 2010. Generally, the population growth rates for Cape Coast since 1970 have been far lower than both the national urban growth rate and the general population growth rate (Ghana Statistical Service, 2010).

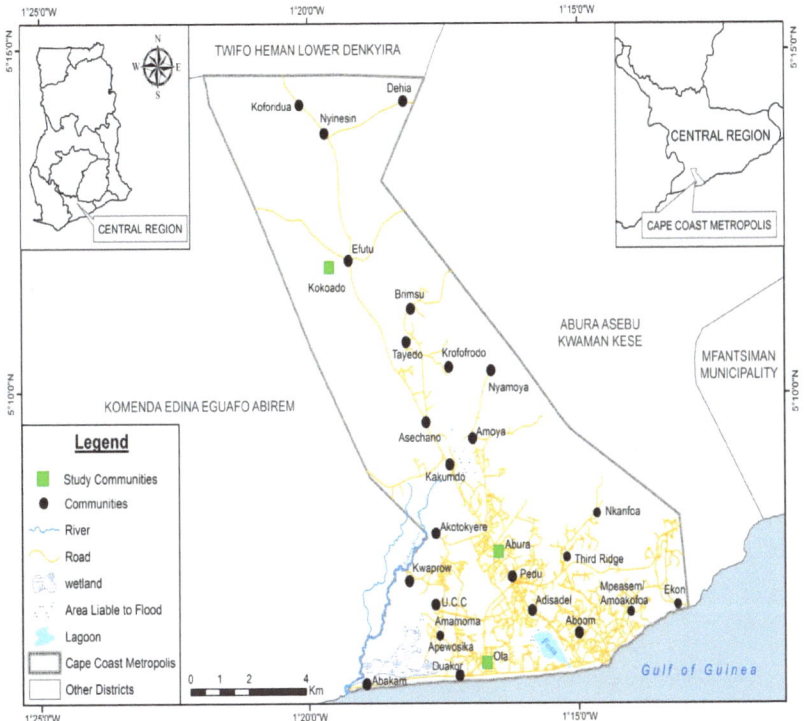

Figure 2: Map of Cape Coast Metropolitan Area showing the study area

Source: Department of Geography and Regional Planning, U.C.C, 2014.

According to Kendie (1998) the low population growth rate of the Metropolis results from out-migration of people from Cape Coast. He further pointed out that the low population growth rate cannot be attributed to fertility decline. Low population growth rate according to Ghana Statistical Service (2010) has produced a high dependency ratio which in the face of few opportunities for employment entrenches poverty.

Undoubtedly, this problem of poverty has severe consequences for environmental sanitation of the area. The Metropolis, which occupies an area of 1700 square kilometres, is made up of 79 settlements. In 2010 the Metropolis had a total population of 169,894 comprising 8, 2810 males (48.7%) and 8, 7084 females (51.3%) with a growth rate of 1.4 per cent (Ghana Statistical Service, 2010).

A large drifting student's population due to existence of many educational institutions and a seasonal arrival of tourist add to the problem of insanitary conditions in the metropolis (Addo, 2010). The facilities that drive people to the metropolis include nine (9) Senior High Schools, one (1) Technical Institute, a Polytechnic, a Teacher Training College, two (2) Nursing Training Colleges and a University (Addo, 2010). There is one castle in the Metropolis that reflects the historical development of this country and which is classified by UNESCO as world heritage monuments. Increasing population compounds the issue of adequate sanitation. The student population adds up to about 25, 000 people to the Metropolis' own population of 169,894 (Ghana Statistical Service, 2010).

Geographical location

The Metropolis is located 145 kilometers west of Accra and 84 kilometers, east of Takoradi. It is bordered to the south by the Gulf of Guinea and to the north by Twifo Heman-Lower Denkyira District and to the west by Komenda-Edina-Eguafo-Abirem District and to the east by Abura-Asebu-Kwamankese District.

Topography

With its location, the Metropolis experiences relatively high temperatures throughout the year. The high temperature, coupled with the high relative humidity means increased rate of decomposition. Under such conditions delayed disposal of waste which in most cases is highly organic in nature has a devastating effect on the quality of air and ultimately on health status of residents.

However, if public waste containers are emptied every day, health effects that solid waste poses to residents will reduce in the metropolis. In addition, the undulating nature of the topography of Cape Coast Metropolis makes the spread of waste management facilities difficult. This has made those residents who cannot access the facilities litter indiscriminately without thinking about the health problems involved.

Waste generation and disposal

The Metropolis is divided into south and north, most of the high and middle income areas are located at the southern part of the Metropolis whereas northern part comprises low income areas of the Metropolis. The northern part of the Metropolis is deprived of adequate sanitation facilities. Inadequate awareness of residents in the northern sector of the Metropolis on how to dispose of waste properly has led to spilling of waste, making the sanitary sites messy and untidy (CCMA-DESSAP, 2009). It is evident that development of the Metropolis is somehow being concentrated in the south at the expense of the north.

A total of 31 health facilities are located in the Metropolis. Of these, 13 are public facilities and 18 are private. Majority of the health facilities are distributed throughout the southern part of the Metropolis, while only one Health Centre is located at Efutu. The northern part of the Metropolis is thus deprived of health facilities.

Research design

Research design is a plan for conducting research which usually includes specification of the elements to be examined and the procedure to be used (Agbesinyale & Anoff 2010). Research design helps to seek information and analyze the evidence of research and also helps to answer initial questions as unambiguously as possible. The study employed a cross sectional study design.

Target population

The study targeted any adult resident aged eighteen (18) years and above because they were matured enough to make meaningful contribution to solid waste issues and respond to questions pertaining to people's perception solid waste disposal in the Metropolis.

Sample size

Sample size answers basic questions such as how large or small must the sample be for it to be representative (Sarantakos, 1998). Choosing the right sample size is a major issue that often confronts social investigators (Creswell, 2003). This study adopted the Fisher, Laing, Stoeckel and Townsend (1998) formula for determining sample size. The formula is given as;

$$n = \frac{z^2 pq}{d^2}$$

Where:

n= the desired sample size (when the population is greater than 10,000);

z= the standard normal deviate, usually set at 1.96 which corresponds to 95 percent confidence level;

p= the proportion in the target population estimated to have particular characteristics;

q= 1.0-p; and

d= degree of accuracy desired, usually set at 0.05.

The sample size (n) for the three communities (OLA, Abura & Kokoado) was found to be as follows:

$$n = \frac{(1.96)^2 \, (0.66) \, (0.28)}{0.05^2}$$

The estimated sample size (n) obtained from the above calculation is two hundred and eighty-four (284) household respondents.

Sampling procedure

The Cape Coast Metropolitan Assembly comprises five (5) zonal councils, these are: Efutu-Kokoado-Mpeasem; OLA-University-Duakor; Abura/Pedu; Aboom-Bakano and Amanful-Ntsin zonal councils. Based on the Ghana Statistical Service demarcation, the study area was stratified into low, middle, and high income areas. Efutu-Kokoado-Mpeasem and Amanful zones represent the low income areas, Aboom-Bakano and Abura/Pedu zones represent middle income areas and OLA-University-Duakor zone represent the high income areas in the Metropolis.

The data was collected from three communities, one from each of the income strata. Based on the distribution of the population of the Cape Coast Metropolis, 284 respondents were proportionately divided among the three communities that were chosen. In each of the selected community, a proportion of 92, 142, and 50 houses were selected from OLA, Abura and Kokoado respectively.

The study employed a range of sampling techniques including stratified, simple random and systematic. The first stage involved zoning of the Metropolis into five zones in line with Cape Coast Metropolitan Assembly's zonal council demarcations. The five demarcated zones were "Zone A, which includes villages in the North-western reaches of the metropolis from

Nyinasen to Kakomdo. This zone represents the predominantly farming communities in the metropolitan area. Zone B consists of communities along the Cape Coast–Jukwa road from Ayifua through Abura to Bakano. Zone C is made up of all communities along the coast from Ekon to OL.A which represents the fishing communities in the metropolis. Zone D is made up of all satellite communities from Apewosika through the University of Cape Coast and Kwaprow to Nkanfua and the ridges. This zone represents a mix bag of high-class residential areas and largely working class and farming villages. Zone E covers the Mfantsipim, Kotokuraba and Tantri areas, which are the commercial sector of the Cape Coast Metropolis. The five zones were further stratified into low, middle and high income areas. This was to get adequate representation and uniformity.

The second stage involved selection of communities. Simple random sampling method was used to select one community from each stratum to represent each of the income categories of the metropolis. This was done by writing the names of all the communities of the income category of the metropolis on pieces of paper and one community was randomly selected. Thus, OLA (high income category), Abura (middle income category) and Kokoado (low income category) were selected to represent the three income categories.

The third stage involved selection of the houses from each of the selected community. Two hundred and eighty four (284) residents aged 18 years and above were selected from the three selected communities. This was done using a systematic sampling technique. Systematic sampling technique was used to choose a house at specific intervals from an ordered arrangement until the sample size was achieved from each of the income category. The number that was assigned to each house in the selected communities formed the sampling frame. The first step was to determine the sampling interval (i). The total number of houses (N) was divided by the sample size (x), that is (i) = N/x. The first ten houses were numbered; the numbers were repeated on pieces of papers and were folded.

One of the folded pieces of paper was randomly selected and number picked represented the first house to be visited. The remaining houses were selected from positions in the sampling frame obtained by adding multiples of "i" to the number drawn by the lottery method. Therefore, 2nd house position is at (K+i)th position, 3rd (K+2i) position, 4th (K+3i)th position. Where "K" is the position of the first house selected from the sampling frame. Every"9th" house was selected until the proportion of each community was covered.

The last stage involved selection of households. One respondent was selected in each house. In houses where there were more than one household, the household were numbered and the same numbers were written on pieces of papers' and folded. One of the folded papers was randomly selected and the person whose number was picked represents the respondent for that house. In cases where only one household is in a house, it was automatically selected. The table below illustrates the sample sizes for each community.

Table 1: Summary of sampling procedures

Communities	2000 Population	Houses	Proportional Allocation	Systematic sampling (n^{th})
OLA	9,938	939	94	9th
Abura	15,326	1,482	140	9th
Kokoado	1,386	204	50	9th
Total	26650	2625	284	

Source of data

The researcher used primary data for the study. Primary data was collected from the three (3) communities in the Cape Coast Metropolis.

Research instrument

Detailed questionnaire was used to collect data from respondents. Those who could read and write were allowed to respond to the questionnaire without support while those who could not read and write were supported. The questionnaire was divided into five sections; section A focused on the demographic characteristics of respondents. Section B also dealt with residents' disposal practices. Moreover, section C looked at residents' attitudes towards solid waste disposal. Section D dealt with residents' perception of solid waste disposal and finally section E focused on the residents' perceived health implications of solid waste disposal. Both open and close ended forms of questions were asked. The choice of the instrument was because of its inherent advantages of it being less expensive over other tools such as focus group discussion and observation (Sarantakos, 1998).

Questionnaire enabled the researcher to obtain data from respondents of the selected communities. Due to the complex nature of disposal and collection of solid waste in the Metropolis the use of quantitative technique (questionnaire) enhanced the chances of getting a more reliable data and minimised the chances of biased findings.

Administration of instruments

Three (3) research assistants who fluently spoke Fante, were recruited for the study. They were taken through a two-day training for the data collection. The training period looked at the purpose of the study and the translation of the instrument into Fante. The researcher with the research assistants pretested the data collection instrument at Moree on the 20th December, 2013. This is because Moree shares similar characteristics with the study communities to assess the suitability of the questions. Twenty (20) residents took part in the trial administration of the questionnaires. The purpose of the pre-testing was to see the realities in administering the instrument and identify possible challenges that could be faced.

The researcher together with research assistants embarked on a reconnaissance survey to the study communities before the actual field work on 1st January to 31st January, 2014. The initial visit provided the opportunity for the researcher to seek permission from chiefs of the selected communities and observe the arrangements of houses in the communities. After the visit, the questionnaires were administered.

Some residents showed unwillingness to partake in the study because they perceived the researchers as sanitary inspectors (asaman-saman) coming from The Cape Coast Metropolitan Assembly to summon them. But the objectives and the purpose of the research were explained to the respondents.

Data analysis

The data were collated and analyzed using software programme; Statistical Product for Service Solutions (SPSS, version 17). Data were analyzed using descriptive statistics. Frequency tables were constructed for the questionnaire items in line with the objectives of the study as an initial step in the analysis. The frequency tables on the demographic variables were constructed as a way of describing the sample population. Cross tabulation tables were also constructed for all multiple response questionnaire items in an attempt to reduce analysis-output and thereby creating compact results of manageable proportions.

Ethical consideration

Ethics means conforming to accepted standards and being consistent with agreed principles of correct moral conduct (Strydom, De Vos, Fouche & Del port, 2005). Informed consent was sought from the respondents before selecting respondents for the data collection. This was achieved by explaining the purpose of the study to the respondents . The purpose was to guarantee free willingness of respondents to participate in the study. Respondents were made aware that information given would be confidentially kept and not exposed to individuals or groups who are not expected to have access to it. Their names and other demographic characteristics such as house numbers that identify them personally were not captured on the questionnaires.

CHAPTER FOUR
RESULTS AND DISCUSSION

Introduction

This chapter presents the findings of the study which are presented under the following sub-headings: socio-demographic characteristics of respondents, residents' solid waste disposal practices, residents' attitudes towards solid waste disposal, residents' perceptions towards solid waste disposal and residents' perceived health implications associated with improper solid waste disposal.

Demographic Characteristics of Respondents

Demographic characteristics of respondents which include place of residence, sex, age and level of education were sought. The results are presented in Table 2. The rationale was to identify the socio-demographic characteristics of the respondents in the selected communities and its influence on residents' solid waste disposal and the perceived health implication related to refuse disposal practices.

Table 2: Background Characteristics of Respondents

Background characteristics	Frequency	Percentage (%)
Sex		
Male	89	31.3
Female	195	68.7
Total	**284**	**100.0**
Age		
15-19	49	17.2
20-24	58	20.4
25-29	60	21.1
30-34	30	10.6
35-39	34	12

40-44	9	3.2
45-49	12	4.2
50-54	8	2.8
55-59	13	4.6
60 and above	11	3.9
Total	**284**	**100.0**

Place of residence

OLA	92	32.4
Abura	142	50
Kokoado	50	17.6
Total	**284**	**100.0**

Level of education

None	25	8.8
Basic	130	45.8
Secondary	74	26.1
Tertiary	55	19.4
Total	**284**	**100.0**

Monthly income

None	38	13.4
Less than 50	26	9.2
50-100	77	27.1
101-200	60	21.1
201-300	17	6.0
301 – 400	16	5.6
>400	50	17.6
Total	**284**	**100.0**

Source: Fieldwork, 2014

Out of the 284 respondents, females constituted the majority (69.0%). The age of respondents ranged from 15 to 60 years and above. Respondents within the age cohorts 20-24 are 20.4 per cent while those within 15-19 and 35-39 years constitute 17.2 per cent and 12 per cent respectively. This indicates that majority of the respondents involved in solid waste disposal in the study area are between 20-24.

Disposal practices among residents

Several solid waste disposal practices have evolved over the years (Centre for Environment and Development, 2003). These practices vary greatly with type of wastes and local conditions. For this reason, the study sought to find out how residents dispose of their solid waste in their various communities. The result is shown in Table 2.

Table 3: Residents disposal practices

Disposal method	Frequency	Percentage
Dump in a skip	162	57.0
Burn it	63	22.2
Door-to-door collection	24	8.5
Dump on the street	22	7.7
Throw it anywhere	13	4.6
Total	284	100.0

Source: Fieldwork, 2014

From Table 2, it is realized that more than half of the respondents (57.0%) indicated they dump their solid waste in a skip that have been provided by CCMA, whereas 4.6 % which constitute about 5.0 per cent of respondents pointed out that they throw their refuse anywhere. This is in line with findings by Yoada et al. (2010) which observed that majority of respondents (61%) dispose their waste in skips that have been provided by the municipal authority.

In order to find out how respondents' perceptions on solid waste disposal are influenced by the community in which they live, the study asked respondents to indicate their place of residence to appreciate the solid waste disposal situation in the selected communities. Table 4 summarizes the result.

Table 4: Residents' solid waste disposal practices by place of residence

	Place of residence		
Disposal practices	OLA	Abura	Kokoado
Burn it	11.0	34.0	10.0
Dump it in a nearby skip	62.0	37.0	66.0
Dump it on the street	2.0	8.0	16.0
Throw it anywhere	14.0	16.0	8.0
Door to door	11.0	5.0	- -
Total	100.0%	100.0%	100.0%

$\chi2 = 26.505$ P-value $= 0.001$ a $= 0.05$
Source: Fieldwork, 2014

While the majority (62.0%) of respondents from OLA said they dump their refuse in a nearby skip, 11.0 per cent said they burn their refuse. Again 2.0 per cent said they dump their refuse on the street as against 11.0 per cent who said they practice door-to-door refuse collection, where 14.0 per cent indicated that they throw their refuse anywhere.

On the other hand, 34.0 per cent of respondents from Abura said they burn their refuse while 37.0 per cent said they dump their refuse in a nearby skip. Eight per cent of respondents from Abura again said they dump their refuse on the street while 16.0% said they throw their refuse anywhere. Again, 5.0 per cent said they practice door- to-door refuse collection.

Moreover, 66.0 per cent of respondents from Kokoado said they dump their refuse in a nearby skip while 10.0 per cent said they burn their refuse. Sixteen and eight per cent again said they dump their refuse on the street and throw their refuse anywhere respectively. This confirms a study by Yoada et al (2014) that most residents dispose their waste in skip, due to their inability to afford the cost house-to-house waste collection service. A chi-square test set at 0.05 produced a p-value of 0.001, indicating a significant relationship between place of residence and solid waste disposal by residents ($\chi2 = 26.505$ P-value $= 0.001$).

In order to ascertain respondents' views on effective ways of dealing with solid waste, respondents were asked to indicate from options provided, the effective way that will be suitable to the metropolis. Table 5 summarises the results.

Table 5: Residents' view on effective way of dealing with solid waste

Disposal practices	Frequency	percentage %
Composting	82	29.0
Burying	56	19.0
Recycling	46	16.0
Land filling	42	15.0
Indiscriminate dumping	33	12.0
Incineration	25	9.0
Total	**284**	**100.0**

Source: Fieldwork, 2014

The results from Table 5 reveal that 29.0 per cent of the respondents indicated that composting of solid waste was an effective way of dealing with waste. This was followed by burying (19.0%), recycling (16.0%), landfilling (15.0%), indiscriminating dumping (12.0%) and incineration (9.0%). Findings on incineration also confirms observation by Gyankumah (2004) that incineration is the least preferred method of dealing with solid for most low-income countries due to its financial requirement.

Table 6: Effective way of dealing with solid waste by place of residence

Solid waste disposal practices	OLA (%)	Abura (%)	Kokoado (%)	Frequency Total	Percentage
		Place of residence			
Incineration	49.0	37.0	14.0	43	100.0
Composting	24.0	69.0	7.0	54	100.0
Landfilling	48.0	19.0	33.0	42	100.0
Recycling	48.0	24.0	28.0	46	100.0
Indiscriminate dumping	9.0	84.0	7.0	33	100.0
Burying	20.0	64.0	16.0	66	100.0
Total				284	100.0

$\chi2 = 66.9$ P-value $= 0.000$ $\alpha = 0.05$

Source: Fieldwork, 2014

How residents deal with solid waste in the metropolis required the study to find out what the residents in the selected communities think is an effective way of dealing with solid waste. It can be observed from Table 6 that out of 92 respondents in OLA 48 per cent indicated recycling to be the most effective way of dealing with solid waste. However, in Abura 84 per cent of the respondents identified indiscriminate dumping as the most effective way of disposing of solid waste. The results on indiscriminate dumping confirms a study by Nabila et al. 1993 which observed that in Ghana about 83 percent of Ghanaians practice indiscriminate dumping. This may be attributed to the cost involve in disposing solid waste by door to door waste collecting system.

Thirty-three per cent of the respondents in Kokoado indicated landfilling as the most effective way of dealing with solid waste. This is in contrast with findings by Addo (2010) that low income communities resort to burying and indiscriminate dumping as their effective way of dealing with solid waste. A chi-square test set at 0.05 produced a p-value of 0.000 indicating a significant relationship between place of residence and effective ways of dealing with solid waste ($\chi2 = 66.9$).

Education is a vital tool for any nation, community as well as the individual. Education usually influences disposal practices of people. Respondents' ways of dealing with solid waste was explored by their level of education. The result is shown in Table 7.

Table 7: Perception of effective way of dealing with solid waste by education

Effective way of dealing with solid waste

Level of Education	Incineration	Composting	Landfilling	Recycling	Indiscriminate dumping	Burying
No education	4.0	6.0	7.0	9.0	15.0	21.0
Basic	47.0	54.0	26.0	39.0	57.0	45.0
Sec./Voc. Technical	27.0	19.0	38.0	24.0	24.0	26.0
Tertiary	22.0	21.0	21.0	28.0	3.0	8.0
Total	100.0%	100.0%	100.0%	100.0%	100.0%	100.0%

$\chi2 = 20.65$

Source: Fieldwork, 2014

From Table 7, 45.0 per cent of the respondents who perceived burying as an effective way of dealing with solid waste had obtained basic education while 8.0 per cent had completed tertiary education. The main reason given by the respondents for suggesting that burying is the most effective method of waste disposal was that, it is the cheapest of all the methods. According to these respondents, solid waste if buried properly does not pose any environmental and health problems. This shows that those who have had basic education though may have had adequate information and knowledge on solid waste disposal and its environmental and health related effects, perhaps do not know the health problems involved in burying solid waste in the communities. This is exemplified in the Pred's Behavioural model matrix conceptual framework for this study where the individual may utilise information optimally based on the quality of information they have (Pred, 1967).

The majority of respondents (57.0 %) with basic education indicated crude dumping as an effective method of disposing waste. The reason cited was because there were limited solid waste facilities in their communities. A chi–square test run produced a p-value of 0.418 indicating a no significant relationship between level of education and effective ways of dealing with solid waste ($\chi2 = 20.65$ P-value = 0.418 a = 0.05).

Best solid disposal practice

The best solid disposal practice is to store domestic in a covered bins. Yoada et al 2014, in their study pointed out that the use of covered bins protects the waste from direct exposure to flies, vermin, scavengers and odour nuisances. Centre for Environment Development (2003) also noted that landfilling, incineration, recycling and composting were the best disposal practices that have evolved over the years. From the study it was realised that 70 percent of respondents cited composting as the best disposal practice. This is in line with the findings put forward by Mensa (2011) that developing countries prefer composting as the best disposal practice.

Residents' attitude towards solid waste disposal

Attitude is an enduring predisposition towards a particular aspect of one's environment (McDougal & Munro, 1987 as cited in Mariwah 2010). The Theory of Planned Behaviour indicates that people's attitude informs their behaviour as well as intention to put up a practice (proper solid waste disposal). For this reason, the study formulated questions to establish residents' attitude on solid waste disposal.

To find out how respondents are involved in solving improper solid waste disposal situation in their communities, they were asked whether they were worried about the solid waste situation in their community or not.

From the study it was revealed that (76.0%) of the residents said they are worried about the way solid wastes are disposed in their environment, (20.0%) said they are not worried, and (4.0%) said they are indifferent about the manner in which solid waste is disposed. It was observed that majority of the residents were worried about the solid waste situation. This confirms assertion by Sessa et al. (2009) that most people are much concerned about improper solid waste issues in their communities.

The issue of whose responsibility it is to keep proper solid waste disposal has become a contention between residents and Metropolitan Assembly nowadays (Franduah, 2008). In order to change people's attitude towards solid waste disposal, it is suggested that the people should be educated to become aware of the problems associated with improper solid waste disposal and see it as a shared responsibility of both the individual and Metropolitan Assembly. The study sought the opinion of respondents on

whose responsibility it is to ensure proper solid waste disposal; the results
is shown in Table 8.

Table 8: Opinions on responsibility for ensuring proper solid waste disposal

Response	Frequency	Percentage (%)
CCMA	131	46.0
Individuals	51	18.0
Both CCMA & individuals	102	36.0
Total	**284**	**100.0**

Source: Fieldwork, 2014

From Table 8, (46.0%) of respondents indicated that the Cape
Coast Metropolitan Assembly is responsible for ensuring proper solid waste
disposal, it is likely that most residents in the study area may not support
clean up campaigns for making the surroundings clean. Furthermore, the
analysis show that 18 per cent of the total respondents thought it was
appropriate for individuals to take the responsibility of ensuring proper solid
waste disposal. Respondents' place of residence was explored by their
perception on whose responsibility is it to collect solid waste in their
community. Seventy per cent of respondents in Kokoado were in support of
the view that the collection of solid waste is the duty of the Metropolitan
Assembly.

This confirms a study in Accra by Franduah (2008) which observed that
residents in Nima are of the view that the Accra Metropolitan Assembly
should be solely responsible for managing solid waste issues in Accra.

Residents' perception on solid waste disposal in their communities

Perception involves the action of our sense organs (sight, hearing, touch, taste, and smell) in responding to external stimulation (Gibson & Tierney, 2006). The Theory of Planned Behaviour explains behavioural beliefs as beliefs about the likely outcomes of the behaviour and the evaluations of these outcomes (Ajzen, 2002).

The issue of what is a problem varies from person to person. Respondents were asked whether they agree or disagree that it is the responsibility of the metropolitan Assembly to provide free dustbin for solid waste collection and disposal to individual homes in the Metropolis.

Residents' perception on the free distribution of dustbins in their communities

The results reveal that 69 per cent of the respondents agreed that the Metropolitan Assembly should provide free dustbin for solid waste in their houses. This may explain why some residents in the study area dump solid waste indiscriminately. They expect the Metropolitan Assembly to provide dustbin in their houses.

It was again observed that about 70 per cent of respondents in all communities studied agreed that Metropolitan Assembly should be responsible for providing free dustbins.

Eighty per cent of the respondents agreed that it was a bad practice to litter around when there is no dustbin. This may mean that some section of the respondents still have negative perception on solid waste disposal and there is the need to educate these group of people on the health effect of indiscriminate solid waste disposal.

Health implications of solid waste disposal

There are several health concerns from improper handling of solid waste (Alam&Ahmade, 2013). Okechukwu, Okechukwu, Noye-Nortey and Owusu-Agyei (2012) stated that due to poor disposal of solid waste, the environmental quality has been affected with prevalent cases of sanitation related diseases such as cholera, typhoid and malaria.

The study investigated respondents' perception on health effect of improper solid waste disposal. The result is shown in Figure 3.

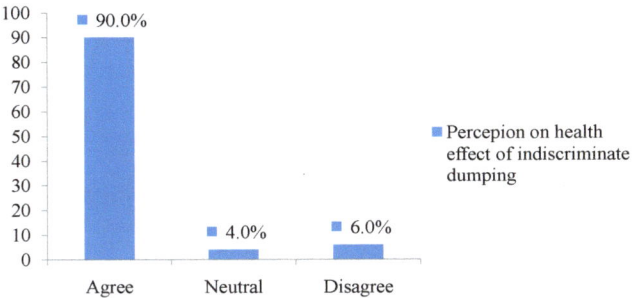

Figure 4: Respondents' perception of effects of improper solid waste disposal on health

Source: Fieldwork, 2014

From Figure 3, 90 per cent of the respondents agreed that people might fall sick if wastes are disposed indiscriminately. This support the findings of Mosquera-Becerra, Gomera-Gutierrez and Mendez-paz (2009) that people in the developing countries hold positive perception that improper solid waste disposal result in negative health outcomes.

Further, respondents were asked their knowledge in relation to health effects of poor solid waste disposal. Eighty-two per cent of respondents were aware of the health implication of poor solid waste disposal. Knowledge of diseases in relation to poor solid waste disposal by respondents includes. Thirty per cent of the respondents said poorly disposed waste promotes the breeding of disease causing germs which could impede health. This is direct consonance with Mizpah and Jay (2009) assertion that poor solid waste disposal present health challenges such as malaria, cholera, cancer and low birth weight. However, 12 percent of the respondents were of the view that evil spirits cause diseases which are commonly known to be sanitation related.

It became necessary to find out perception of respondents on solid waste disposal by place of residence due to the fact that most residents have different perceptions on solid waste disposal and its health effect.

Eighteen per cent of the respondents in Kokoado and 12.0 per cent of the respondents in Abura were in support that their body is used to dirt and as a result the dirty environment cannot make them sick. Whereas 88.0 per cent of the respondents in Abura disagreed to the statement. This confirms a study in Cape Coast by Kendie (1998) which observed that residents in Adisadel do not agree that dirty environment cannot make them sick.

A chi – square test run show a significant relationship between place of residence and my body is used to dirt (p-value, 0.000).

Perceived health problems associated with solid waste disposal

Health problems associated with sanitation are normally perceived differently by different people. As such, what may appear to be sanitation-related diseases also differ by contexts and persons Table 9 illustrates their responses.

Table 9: Respondents' perception on health problems associated with solid waste disposal by percentage

Diseases	SA	A	N	D	SD
	%	%	%	%	%
Malaria	75.0	17.0	2.0	4.0	2.0
Cholera	88.0	11.0	1.0	-	-
Typhoid	59.0	10.0	17.0	6.0	7.0
Dysentery	57.0	11.0	21.0	5.0	7.0
Diarrhoea	71.0	15.0	7.0	6.0	1.0
* R.T.I	48.0	13.0	20.0	5.0	14.0

* Respiratory Tract Infection

SA= strongly agree A= agree N= neutral D= disagree and SD= strongly disagree

Source: Fieldwork, 2014

From Table 9, almost all the respondents agreed that cholera is associated with improper solid wastes disposal. The majority 92 percent agreed malaria is associated with poor wastes disposal. Again, about 86.0 per cent agreed that diarrhoea is associated with improper wastes disposal. Moreso, 69 percent agreed that typhoid was associated with improper solid wastes disposal in the community. This confirms the statistics from the Epidemiological Department of Ministry of Health (2013) which reveals that malaria, diarrhoea and cholera are incidence of sanitation related diseases among the top ten morbidity O.P.D cases within the metropolis.

Moreover, the findings of Mizpah and Jay (2009) agree with the result that disposal of solid waste without careful planning and management can present a danger to the environment and diseases such as malaria, cholera and diarrhoea to people. It again confirms a study by Yoada et al (2014) that more than half (84%) of respondents in Medina were aware that improper solid waste disposal leads to sickness.

CHAPTER FIVE
SUMMARY, CONCLUSIONS AND RECOMMENDATIONS

Introduction

This final chapter presents the summary, conclusions and recommendations based on the findings. Whereas the summary gives a brief overview of the research problem, objective, methodology and findings; the conclusions capture the overall outcomes regarding the findings of the study in light of the research questions. The recommendations also present specific remedies to be implemented by specific bodies.

Summary

The study was undertaken to assess residents' perception of solid waste disposal in the Cape Coast Metropolis. The study aimed to identify solid waste disposal practices of residents; assess attitudes of residents towards solid waste disposal; analyse the perception of residents on solid waste disposal and discuss the perceived health implications of disposal of solid waste disposal.

A cross section research design was adopted.the design helped to answer the research questions as unambiguously as possible and also examines the situation as it exists in its current state. The study used the questionnaire to illicit or collect information from the respondents. The study was carried out in three communities in the Cape Coast Metropolis. The communities were OLA, Abura and Kokoado. A total of 284 respondents were used for the study. A multi-stage sampling was used to select the respondents.

Again the study used the SPSS programme to analyse the data. Some of the variables were subjected to statistical tests with a view to finding statistical significance of association where applicable. This was to make well informed and reliable analysis for acceptable and reliable conclusions to be drawn.

From the objectives it was realised that:

Forty-two per cent of the respondents were within the age cohort 20-29 and the majority of them were females (69.0%). About forty-six per cent (45.8) were basic school graduate while 27.1 per cent of the respondents earned an average of GH¢100 per month.

It was revealed that 57 percent of the respondents dump their solid waste in a skip and quite a few 8 percent throw theirs on the streets. It was also found that whereas 22 per cent of the respondents in all the communities indicated they burn their solid waste and 5 per cent said they throw their solid waste anywhere.

Moreover on solid waste disposal practice, most of respondents mentioned composting, burying and recycling of wastes as some of the effective ways of disposing waste. In terms of place of residence, it was significant that 48 percent, 49 percent and 24 percent people at OLA mentioned recycling, incinerating and compositing respectively, perhaps they probably have knowledge in them.

It was identified that 76.0 per cent of the respondents were worried about the improper handling of solid waste and 46.0 per cent of them were those in the high income area. Again 46.0 per cent of the respondents expressed the opinion that the onus lies on the Cape Coast Metropolitan Assembly to ensure proper solid waste disposal.

It was ascertained that most of these improper handling of wastes in the areas give rise to other diseases like malaria, cholera, typhoid, diarrhoea and other respiratory tract diseases.

Conclusions

The study empirically examined the perception of people on the effects of solid waste in the Cape Coast metropolis. From the findings all the objectives were accomplished. Though the majority 57 percent of the respondents said they throw their solid waste into a nearby waste bins, about 8 percent of the respondents throw solid waste on the streets. It appears that most of these respondents who said they throw their solid waste onto the street were people from the middle income category. Again a lot of the respondents stated composting as a proper way of dealing with solid waste without recourse to the money and veracity of expertise needed.

The study found a significant relationship between place of residence of respondents and disposal practices they think was appropriate. Most of the respondents at OLA indicated recycling and composting of solid waste. This may possibly mean because they could afford the fees that would be charged in such case and the consequences on the other practices. On the other hand, those in the middle and low income areas stated burning, burying and landfilling of solid waste perhaps it was cheap. It could also be concluded that those respondents with higher level of education and also knowledgeable of the ramifications of burning, landfilling and indiscriminate dumping of waste hinted that the proper ways of dealing with solid waste was to recycle or composite them.

For the attitude of respondents, most respondents (76%) expressed worries over the improper disposal of waste and most affected were those found to be in the high income category. Respondents however expressed the opinion that the assembly (CCMA) and the individuals should share the responsibility of ensuring proper disposing of solid in their surroundings regarding the worries at the backdrop of their minds. Also, majority of respondents expect the CCMA to provide free dustbin for them in their houses. This could explain why some residents in the study practiced

66

improper solid waste disposal. However, majority of respondents agreed that it was a bad practice to litter around when there is no dustbin. Almost all the respondents irrespective of their area of settlement agreed that indiscriminately dumping of waste possess a threat to health and not rather evil spirits. Majority of respondents were aware that improper solid waste disposal leads to sickness. Respondents mentioned that the health risk involved were malaria, cholera, typhoid, diarrhoea and other respiratory tract infections.

Recommendations

Based on the key findings of the study the following recommendations are made :

1. The Cape Coast Metropolitan Assembly in collaboration with the Ministry of Health should intensify education on the dangers of indiscriminate dumping of solid waste annually.

2. The Assembly (CCMA) should also provide a number of waste bins at vantage areas in the various communities. The low and middle income communities should be supplied with enough containers to avoid indiscriminate dumping of waste in gutters, open spaces, streets and nearby bushes.

3. There should be public education on proper ways of solid waste disposal in the metropolis to inform the general public on the implications of unhealthy environment and the need to keep their communities clean. The education could be done by Zoomlion and the Environmental Health Department of the Cape Coast Metropolitan Assembly.

Areas for further research

The current study focused on residents' perceptions of solid waste disposal in the Cape Coast Metropolis. Further studies can be undertaken to look at the service providers (Zoomlion and CCMA) perceptions on solid waste disposal.

Detailed study in health implications of improper solid waste disposal will pave way for residents to appreciate and understand the need to keep clean environment.

REFERENCES

Abagale, K. F., Mensah, A. & Agyemang-Osei, R. (2012). Urban solid waste sorting in a growing city of Ghana. *International Journal of Environment and Sustainabilty, 1* (4), 18 -25.

Achor, P.N., Ehikwe, A. A., & Nwafor, A. U.(2014). Curbing/Mitigating indiscriminate waste dumping through effective stakeholder relations. *International journal of science and research*,*1*, 2319-7064.

Abduli, A. & Nasrabadi, T. (2007). Municipal solid waste management in Kurdistan province, Iran. *Journal of Hetillfi, 69* (7), 51-55.

Abul, S. (2010). Environmental and health impact of solid waste disposal at Mangwaneni dumpsite in Manzini, Swaziland. *Journal of Sustainable Development in Africa, 12*(7), 64-78.

Achankeng, E. (2003). *Globalisation, urbanisation and municipal solid waste management in Africa: Africa on a global stage.* A Paper presented at the Annual Conference of the African Studies Association of Australasia and the   Pacific.

Addo, M. (2010). *Solid waste management practices in the Cape Coast Metropolis*. Unpublished dissertation submitted to institute for development studies, University of Cape Coast, Cape Coast, Ghana.

Adekunle, I. M., Oguns, O., Shekwolo, O., Igbuku, A. O. & Ogunkoya, O. O. (2012). *Assessment of population perception impact on value-added solid waste disposal in developing countries: A case study of Port Harcourt city, Nigeria*. Retrieved November 2013 from http//www.intechopen.com

Afroz, R., Hanaki, K. & Tuddin, R.(2010). The role of socio-economic factors on household waste generation: a study in a waste management program in Dhaka city, Bangladesh. *Research Journal of Applied Sciences. 5*(3),183-190.

Agbesinyale, P. & Anoff, J. (2010). *Notes in research methods*. Cape Coast: University of Cape Coast Press.

Ajzen, I. (2002). Perceived behavioural control, self-efficient, locus of control, and the theory of planned behaviour. *Journal of Applied Social Psychology, 32*, 665-683.

Alam, P. & Ahmade, K. (2013). Impact of solid waste on health and the environment. *International journal of sustainable development and green economics, 2(1)*, 2315-4721.

Appiah, P., Obeng, E., Donkor, A. & Mensah, A. (2009). Assessment of institutional structures for solid waste management in Kumasi. *International Journal, 20*(2), 106-120.

Bandara, N.J., Hettiaratchi, J.P.,Wirasinghe, . S.C. & Pilapiiya, S. (2007). Relation of waste generation and composition to socio-economic factors: a case study. *Environmental Monitoring and Assessment*. 135:31–39.

Banjo, A. D., Adebambo, A. A. R. & Dairo, O. S. (2009).Inhabitants' perception on domestic waste disposal in Ijebu Ode, Southwest Nigeria. *African Journal of Basic and Applied Sciences, 1*(3), 62-66.

Barlaz, M., Kaplan, P., Ranjithan, S. & Rynk, R. (2003). Evaluating environmental impacts of solid waste management alternatives. *Biocycle,* 52-56.

Barnhart, R. K. (2008). *The World book dictionary*, Chicago: World Book Inc. Bartley, S. W. (2009). *Principles of perception*. New York: Harper Row Publishers.

Benneh, G., Songsore, J., Nabila, S.J. Amuzu, A.T. & Tutu, K.A. (1993). *Environmental problem and urban household In Greater Accra Metropolitan Area (GAMA)*. M.A.C. Stockholm, Ghana.

Bernstein, J. (2004). *Social assessment and public participation in municipal solid waste management*. Washington D.C.: Urban Environment Thematic Group, the World Bank.

Boadi, K. O. & Kuitunen, M. (2003). Municipal solid waste management in Accra metropolitan area, Ghana. *The Environmentalist, 23* (3), 211-218.

Bowersox, D. J., Closs, D. J. & Cooper, M. B. (2005). *Supply chain logistics management.* Washington D. C.: McGraw – Hill.

Browne, M. & Allen, J. (2007). *Logistics and waste sector: London case study.* London: Transport studies group,

Cape Coast Metropolitan Assembly-District environmental and sanitation strategy and plan(CCMA-DESSAP) (2009). Retrieved August 2013 from http:// www.ccma.ghanadistrictgov.gh accessed

Centre for Diseases Control (2009). Study of the attitude and perception of community towards solid waste management. Thiruvanathapuram: *Kerala Research Programme on Local Level Development.*

Centre for Environment and Development (2003). *Study of the attitude and perception of community towards solid waste management*. Washington, D. C.: CED.

Chati, T. J. (2012). *Solid waste management in Ghanaian towns: A case of Saboba, Northern region*. Unpublished master's thesis, Kwame Nkrumah University of Science and Technology, Kumasi.

Cointreau, S. J. (2002). Declaration of principles for sustainable and integrated solid waste management. Accessed at:http://web.worldbank.org.on 17/06/07.

Cointreau, S. (1982). *Environmental management of urban solid waste in developing countries: a project guide*. Urban Development Department, World bank.

Coolidge, J.G., Porter, R.C. & Zhang, Z.J. (1998). Urban environmental services in developing countries. Department of Economics, University of Michigan.

Creswell, J.W. (2003). *Research design: Qualitative, quantitative and mixed methods approaches* (2nd Ed). Thousand Oaks, CA: Sage Publication.

Davies, A. R. (2008). *The geographies of garbage governance: Intervention, interactions and outcomes*. London: Ashgate.

Dango, K., Zurbrugg, C., Cisse, B., Tanner, M. & Biemi, J. (2010). Analysing environmental risks and perceptions of risks to assess health and well-being in poor areas of Abidjan. *International Journal of Civil and Environmental Engineering 3, 20-29.*

Danso-Manu, K.B. (2011). *The nature of solid waste management in Ghana: towards data collection for good management practices.* Kumasi: Kwame Nkrumah University of Science and Technology press.

Da-Zhu, P., Asnani, H., Zurbrugg, C., Anapolsky, S. & Mani, S. (2008). *Improving municipal solid waste of existing MSW management in India: A source book for policymakers and practitioners.* Washington D.C.: World Bank.

Department of Geography and Regional Planning (2014). *Map of the study area.* Cartographic Unit, University of Cape Coast.

Dijkema, G. P. J., Reuter, M. A. & Verhoef, E. V. (2000). A new paradigm for waste management. *Waste Management, 20*(8), 633-638.

Dolk, H. (2003). Methodological issues related to epidemiological assessment of health risks of waste management. *Revues Epidem Sante Publique, 53,* 2S87-2S95.

Environmental guidelines for small- scale activities in Africa (EGSAA) (2009) Solid waste generation, handling, treatment and disposal. Washington D.C: USAID.

Fieandt, K. V. (2006). *The world of perception.* Illinois: The Dorsey Press.

Fisher, A. A., Laing, J. E., Stoeckel, J. E. & Townsend, J. W. (1998). Handbook for family planning operations research design. *Waste Management, 20*, 633-638.

Forgus, R. H. (2010). Perception: *The basic process in cognitive development.* New York: McGraw-Hill.

Franduah, G. (2008). *Problem of solid waste management in Nima, Accra.* A dissertation submitted to the department of environmental science University of Ghana, Legon. Retrieved October 2013 from http://www.kon.org/u6/george

Gadsby, A. (Ed.). (2003). *Longman Dictionary of Contemporary English: the living dictionary*. London: Pearson Education Limited.
Ghana Districts. (2013). *Cape Coast profile*. Retrieved August 2013 from www.ccma.ghanadistrictgov.gh

Ghana Statistical Service (2010). *2010 population and housing census report.* Accra: Ghana Statistical Service.
Ghana Health Service (2012). *Central Regional Annual Report 2012*. Cape Coast: Ghana Health Service.

Ghana Statistical Service (2008). *Ghana Living standard survey-5*, Accra: Combert Impression.

Gibson, K. & Tierney, J. K. (2006). Electrical waste management and disposal: Issues and alternatives. *Environmental Claims Journal, 18,* 321-332.

Gladding, T. (2004). *Health risks of materials recycling facilities: Environmental and health impact of solid waste management activities.* Geneva: World Health Organization.

Goorah, S., Esmyot, M. & Boojhawon, R. (2009). The health impact of non-hazardous solid waste disposal in a community: The case of the mare chicose landfill in Mauritius. *Journal of Environment Health, 72* (1), 48-54.

Gyankumah, F. K. (2004). *Management of solid waste in Ghana: Case study of Accra Metropolitan Assembly* Unpublished B.S.C (Planning) Special Study Submitted to the Department of Planning, University of Science and Technology, Kumasi.

Hamdi, N. (2003). 'Small Change: About the Art of Practice and the Limits of Planning in Cities', Earthscan publishing

Hester, R. E. & Harrison, R. M. (Eds.) (2003*). Environmental and health impact of solid waste management activities.* Cambridge: The Royal Society of Chemistry.

Jessen, M. (2002). *Zero waste services.* Retrieved May 2013, from http://www.zerowaste.ca/articles.

Johansson, O. M. (2006). The effect of dynamic scheduling and routing in a solid waste management system. *Waste Management, 26* (8), 875-885.

Kaseva, M. E. & Mbuligwe, S. E. (2003). *Appraisal of solid waste collection following private sector involvement in Dar es Salaam City.* Dodoma*:* Habitat International.

Karley, N.A. (1993). (October, 9, 1993). *Solid Waste and Pollution*. Accra.People's daily graphic.

Kendie, S. B. (1998). Do Attitudes Matter?: Waste disposal and wetland pollution in the Cape Coast Municipality of Ghana. *Malaysian journal of tropical Geography*, *29* (2), 69-81.

Kendie, S. B. (2003). *Linking water supply, sanitation and hygiene in northern Ghana*. Cape Coast: Catholic Mission Press.

Kistner, T. (2005). *Efficient waste management in focus of a logistics provider*. Dautche Post: DHL Solutions.

Kitbuah, E., Asase, M., Yusif, S., Mensah. Y. & Fischer, K. (2009). *Comparative analysis of households waste in the cities of Stuttgart and Kumasi: options for recycling and treatment in Kumasi.* Kumasi. Mission Press.

Longe, E. O., Longe, O. O. & Ukpebor, E. F. (2009). People's perception on household solid waste management in Ojo local government area in Nigeria. *Iran Journal Environment Health Science Engineer, 6*(3), 209-216.

Mariwah, S., Kendie, S. B. & Dei, A. L. (2010). Residents' perception of the solid waste problem in the Shama-Ahanta-East metropolitan area, Ghana. *Oguaa Journal of Social Sciences, 5*, 1.

Markwara, E.C. (2011). Work related environmental health risks: the case of garbage handlers in the city of Masvingo, Scarbrucken, Lambert Academic Publishing.

Maurice, W. (Ed.). (2007). *The New Shorter Oxford English Dictionary*. Sixth Edition. Oxford University Press.

Malombe, J.M. (1993). "Sanitation and Solid Waste Disposal in Malindi, Kenya. 19th*Water, Sanitation, environment and development conference preprints*, Ghana.

Medina, M. (2002). *Globalization, Development and Municipal Solid Waste Management in Third World Cities*. Institute of Advance Studies, Mexico.

Melissa, G. (Ed). (2002). Macmillan English Dictionary for Advanced Learners. *International student edition*. London: Bloomsbury Publishers.

Mazmanian, D. & Kraft, M. (2005). *Toward sustainable communities: Transitions and transformations in environmental policy*. Cambridge: MIT Press.

Mbalisi, O.F. & Offor, B.O. (2012). Imperatives of environmental education and awareness creation to solid waste management in Nigeria. *Journal of Education*, *3*(2), 10-36.

Mensa, E. A. (2011). *Management of solid waste in Kumasi central market*. Kumasi: Kwame Nkrumah University of Science and Technology.

Mensah, A. & Larbi, E. (2005) *Fact sheet; Solid waste disposal in Ghana*. Kumasi: Directorate of Waste Management.

Mills-Tettey, R. (2011). *Geography of sub-Saharan Africa*. Upper Saddle River, N. J: Prentice Hall.

Ministry of Health (2013). *Epidemiological department annual statistical report, Cape Coast.* Cape Coast: Ministry of Health .

Ministry of Local Government and Rural Development (2010). *Environmental sanitation policy.* Accra: MLGRD.

Mizpah, A. & Jay, S. (2009). Comparison of municipal solid waste management system in Canada and Ghana: A case study of the cities London, Ontario and Kumasi, Ghana. *Waste Management 29*, 2779–2786.

Moeller, D. W. (2005). *Environmental Health* (3rd ed.). Cambridge: Harvard University Press.

Mosquera-Becrra, J., Gomez-Gutierrez, O. L. & Mendez-Paz, F. (2009). Impact perception on health, social and physical environments of the municipal solid waste disposal site in Cali. *Review SaludPublica Bogota, 68*(1), 183-197.

Murad, M.W., Hasan, M.M.&Rahman, M.S.(2012). Relationship between personality traits of the urban poor concerning solid waste management and household income and education. *Description of complex systems*, 10(2), 174-192.

Nachmias, C. F. & Nachmias, D. (1996). *Research methods in the social sciences.* Washington, D. C.: Nesttalie Ltd.

NEMA (2012). *National environment management authority*. Retrieved August 2013, from http://www.nema.go.

Njagi, J. M., Ireri, A. M., Njagi, E. N. M., Akunga, D., Afullo, A. T. O., Ngugi., M. P., Mwanzo, I. & Njagi, I. K. (2013). Knowledge , attitude and perceptions of village residents on the health risks posed by Kadhodeki dumpsite in Nairobi, Kenya. *Ethiopian journal of environmental studies and management. (6)* 4, 1-8.

Nze, F.C. (1978). "Managing Urban Waste in Nigeria for Social and economic development" *Journal of Management Studies, 5*(2).

Okechukwu, O. L, Okechukwu, A. A., Noye-Nortey, H. & Owusu-Agyei, J. (2012). Health perception of indiscriminate waste disposal: A Ghanaian case study. *Journal of Medicine and Medical Sciences 3(3*), 146-154.

Olar, Z. (2003). *Urban solid waste management: waste reduction in developing nations.* Michigan: Technological University Press.

Onibokun, A. G. & Kumuyi A. J. (2004). Governance and waste management in Africa. In Onibokun, A. G. (Ed). (2004). Managing the monster. Urban waste and governance in Africa. Canada, International Development

Research Centre (IDRC). www.idrc.ca/publication/onlinebooks on 20/12/13 Palczynski, R. J. (2004). *Study on solid waste management options for Africa.* Wolfville: African Development Bank Sustainable Development and Poverty Reduction Unit.

Poku, O. (2009). *Waste disposal management in the peri-urban areas of Kumasi.* Kumasi: DFID. Retrieved from www.dfid.com.

Porter, R. & Boakye-Yiadom, J. (1997). *The economics of water and waste in three African capitalists*. Ashgate Publishing Limited, England.

Pred, A. (1967). *Behaviour and location*. London, Royal University of London. Roel, G., Eddy, V. V. & Thierry, V. (2010). *Assessing characteristics of waste logistics from an innovation perspective*. Antwerp: University of Antwerp.

Rushbrook, P. & Pugh. S. (1999*).* Solid waste landfills in middle-and lower-income countries. *World Bank Technical Paper, 426*.

Satterthwaite, D. (1998). Enviromental problems in cities in the south: sharing my confusions. In, Fernandes Edesio (ed), *environmental strategies for sustainable development in urban areas. Lessons from Africa and Latin America.* Ashgate Publishing Ltd, England.

Sarantakos, S. (1998). *Social research*. New York: Palgrave Macmillan Limited.

Scheinberg, A, Anschutz, J. & Van de K. A. (2006). *Waste pickers: Poor victims or waste management professionals*. A paper presented at CWG-WASH workshop 2006, 1-5 February in Kolkata, India.

Senkoro, M. (2003). *Solid waste management in Africa: A WHO/AFRO perspective*. Paper presented in Dar Es Salaam at the CWG Workshop.

Retrieved from www.skat.ch/sf web/activities/ws/cwg/pdf/cwg. on 4/11/2013.

Sessa, A., Giuseppe, G., Marinelli, P. & Angelillo, I. (2009). Public concerns and behaviours towards solid waste management in Italy. *The European Journal of Public Health, 4,* 35-49.

Sivakumar, K. & Sugirtharan, M. (2010). Impact of family income and size on per capita solid waste generation: a case study in Manmunai north divisional secretariat division of Batticaloa. *Journal of scicence, 5,* 13-23.
Strategic Environmental Assessment (SEA) of MTDP (2010). *International source book on environmentally sound technologies for municipal solid waste management*. New York: UNEP.

Strydom, H., De Vos, A. S., Fouche, C. B. & Del port, C. S. L. (2005). *Research at grassroots for the social sciences and human service professions*. Pretoria: Van Schalk.

Sule, O. R. A.(1981). "Management of Solid Wastes in Nigeria towards a Sanitary Urban Environment". *Quarterly journal of Administration*, Lagos vol. 15, Nigeria.

Swan, J. R. (2003). *Microbial emissions from composting sites. Environmental and Health Impact of Solid Waste Management Activities*, 73-101.

Taiwo, M. A. (2011). Composting as a sustainable waste management technique in developing countries. *Journal of Environmental Science and Technology, 4* (2), 93-102.

Thrift, C. (2007). *Sanitation policy in Ghana: Key factors and the potential for ecological sanitation solutions*. Stockholm: Stockholm Environmental Institute. Retrieved from www.ecosanres.org.

Tsiboe, I. A. & Marbell, E. (2004*). A look at urban solid waste disposal problem in Accra, Ghana*. Unpublished master's thesis submitted to Roskilde University.

UNEP (2005). *Selection, design and implementation of economic instruments in the solid waste management sector in Kenya*. The case of plastic bags.

New York: Author. Retrieved August 2013 from www.unep.org.
UNEP (2007). *Environmental pollution and impacts on public health: Implications of the Dandora Municipal dumping site in Nairobi*.

United Nations Environmental Programme (2009). *Developing integrated solid waste management plan training manual: Assessment of current waste management system and gaps therein*. Osaka: UNEP.

United Nations Development Programme (UNDP) (2009*). Ghana National Human Development report 2008*, Accra: UNDP.

United Nations Environmental Program (2006). *Marine and coastal ecosystems and human well-being: a synthesis report based on the findings of the millennium ecosystem assessment*. Osaka: UNEP.

United Nations Environmental Program (2012), *developing integrated solid waste management plan training manual. Assessment of current waste management system in developing world and gaps therein*. Osaka: UNEP.

United State Environmental Protection Agency (U.S.E.P.A), (2009). Municipal solid waste in the United States : 2009 facts and figures.

Washington D.C., E.P.A US office of Research and Development.
World Bank (2000). *What a waste! Solid waste management in Asia*.

Washington D. C.: The World Bank.World Health Organisation (2009). *Landfills and solid waste and health: Briefing pamphlets on solid waste.* Copenhagen: WHO.

Yoada, R. M., Chirawurah, D. & Adongo, P. B. (2014). *Domestic waste disposal practice and perceptions of private sector waste management in urban Accra*. 14-697.

www.ingramcontent.com/pod-product-compliance
Lightning Source LLC
Chambersburg PA
CBHW050808290526
45792CB00001B/24